HONOR YOUR JOURNEY

BY
SHIRLEY GILBERT, Ph.D.
All proceeds go toward helping abused animals.

Printed in the United States of America
ISBN: Softcover   978-1-63871-700-3
               eBook   978-1-63871-701-0
Republished by: PageTurner Press and Media LLC
Publication Date: 11/08/2021

To order copies of this book, contact:
PageTurner Press and Media
Phone: 1-888-447-9651
info@pageturner.us
www.pageturner.us

DEDICATION

I love animals, especially dogs. One of my best friends is my very special, loyal, furry friend, Maxwell Smart XXIII (AKC, West Highland Terrier), better known as "Max."

He has been by my side throughout the writing of this book. He has provided love, sloppy kisses, unending patience, and taken me for walks. How blessed I am to have such a little friend to whom I owe a debt of gratitude for the unconditional love he has shown me, and taught me. Max (a registered therapy dog) and I want to help hurting people as well as our many furry hurting friends. Please help us.......

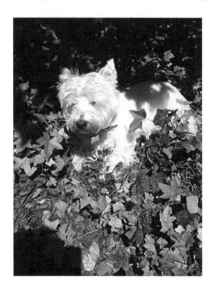

INTRODUCTION

It's all been said.

The challenge to write a self-help book that interests people and motivates them to want to improve their lives is a daunting task, no matter how many degrees or decades of experience one may have, nor how much we may want it to happen.

Nonetheless, this is the motivation behind this book. I write in hopes that my life, education and experiences, and the way I present them, could make a positive difference for someone.

When my career ended suddenly due to an accident in the work place prison, many years ago, I thought long and hard about how I could continue to try to make a difference for good. That desire gave birth to this book.

If your life was to end today, what would be your greatest regret? If you could have one wish granted, what would it be? The answers to these questions give us some idea of our life journey. In fact, this is a book about identifying our best life path and making it a reality. Along our journey, we check out many paths as we seek to find our way.

Are you able to identify that time in your life when you made a decision that provided a definite curve on your life path? Maybe it was one you have since regretted? We have all done that. It doesn't mean we can't get up, dust ourselves off and start again. That's what life requires.

Life has taught me that most of us give up our power at an early age and never take it back. We spend our lives giving it to other people and come to the end of life, never having lived it the way we wanted. We were too busy trying to make others like us, get ahead, make money, keep up with our neighbors, make certain people knew we were important.

My time in Hospice (where people go to die) tells me these are not the values people cling to at the end. Many are heartbroken over not having been the authentic person they are and they have not lived their life on their own terms. Their time for living and choosing has come and gone and they are out of time for making life choices.

Most of them talk about family, where they learned about and felt love, or not. As John Powell says, "Our lives are shaped by those who have loved us and those who have refused to love us." These are the kinds of things people reflect on during their last days.

This is a book about learning life skills that can help us be the best we possibly can. It is a mental health blueprint for living.

We can dream our dreams, put foundations under them and try our best to make them happen. We won't always succeed, but we are always wise to try.

Understanding and gaining insights into building our best life is what this book is about. Read it, dare to believe in yourself and determine to make your life journey your very best. The power is yours to make it happen.

Since my effort is to help people, and honor abused animals, I encourage you to buy several copies for friends and family and recommend it to others. This is a book for everyone.

Shirley Gilbert, Ph.D.

Clinical Psychologist

TABLE OF CONTENTS

Chapter One

MAKING HEALTHY CHOICES

"To thine own self be true, but which self?"
(Dr. Fritz Heider)

We are who we are because that's who we have chosen to be, one choice at a time. We got to where we are, one choice at a time.

The power to choose is one of the greatest human strengths. Taking responsibility for our choices appears to be the hard part. We often attribute the state of our life to others.

There exists a very strong connection between the choices we make, which end up defining who we are, and our capacity to honor our journey.

Clearly, however, there are many choices which are <u>not</u> ours to make. We come into the world with so many things that are out of our control.

Each of us is dealt a different hand. Each of us has a different test, if you will. The goal is to make the best we can of the hand we've been dealt as well as the environment in which we find ourselves.

It is my opinion as a mental health professional that all hands dealt are not equal. Another way of saying that is that life is not always fair. It is true that we can make wise choices and set positive goals for our lives, but much of it is out of our control.

In my professional experience, I have treated the 'worried, well and wealthy,' the hated mass murderer, and the physically, mentally and sexually abused child. Each of them were likely dealt a different hand.

The point I am making here is that people often waste so much of their lives being angry or seriously depressed about the hand they were dealt. It is what it is.

Parents and others are often blamed for these feelings and problems as opposed to taking responsibility for how we feel about ourselves and our lives. If we don't like it, we have the power to make changes.

At some point, however, these facts and feelings need to be accepted and dealt with so people can make the best of the gifts they have.

There are thousands of examples of people with disabilities of all kinds which they have overcome and manage every day. They are examples for us all. They amaze me. I once spent a week at the Mayo Clinic and could hardly believe the resiliency people demonstrated. People are amazing in so many ways.

As we all know, there are many people who come from very wealthy homes, very privileged people who have ruined their chances of a productive life by making bad choices. I am thinking of the children of famous movie stars who are serving time for murder, drugs, sexual violence, DUI's or have suicided.

Life isn't just about the hand we've been dealt, it's all about the choices we make. We've heard that when life gives us lemons, we should make lemonade. I have actually witnessed people who have been able to do exactly that. Others, who have been given so much, throw it away. I've seen that also.

What I have learned personally in my own life as well as in the lengthy years of education and experience is that our choices are what make or break us. We don't have control over many things that happen to us, but we do have control over how we choose to respond to them!

Coping skills are usually developed as a result of having to deal with and find a way to manage pain and problems. We have many choices about how to resolve our issues. Giving up should not be one of them, yet we see thousands of examples of this increasingly.

Some people, not suffering from mental illness, use life as a means of hurting as many others as brutally as possible. Others manage their pain compassionately and use it as a means of helping to alleviate the suffering of others. For both of these people, they are exercising a choice. They have chosen "which self" they want to be.

I believe most of us have no idea of the true power we have by utilizing healthy choices to honor our path. Whatever happened to "kinder and gentler?"

The whole point of honoring our path is that of making healthy choices. That is, in fact, what it means to make healthy choices, to honor the person we have chosen to become.

I have witnessed these diverse paths from children raised in the same family. They have the same parents, same environment, same school, etc. Yet, they are totally diverse. How do we account for that?: choices!

In order to honor our path, we have to respect the person on the path. That is usually the result of having made healthy choices. When we talk about being true to ourselves, even there, we have a choice, "Which self?" My mentor and friend, Dr. Fritz Heider was very creative in taking Shakespeare's famous phrase and reframing it in this insight way. " Which self?" It is up to us to choose.

The ability to block is very central to having mental health. Being able to block is a choice! It's not an easy choice, but, nevertheless, it is a choice. We have tremendous power when we are able to block. That is part of honoring the self we have chosen to become. We need to learn to get out of our feelings and into our head in order to become disciplined to make certain choices, such as the ability to block.

I have found it very helpful to journal as a way of keeping track of myself and my choices. I divide my journaling into three columns: thinking, feeling and doing. That is, what are my thoughts? What are my feelings? How am I acting it all out, i.e., my behavior. I also pay attention to whether or not I am congruent. That is, do my thoughts, feelings and behaviors line up? Or, am I thinking one thing, feeling another and doing another. Human behavior is very complex.

There is so much that goes into making choices. Most people are so busy just trying to make it through the day, they don't often give much thought to making choices or, to be honest, feel as though they even have many choices to control their lives. This is unfortunate. Each person has a unique skill set but often gets caught up in the pressures of everyday life and never pays attention to their uniqueness.

I believe that a very big part of stress management is staying focused on our ability to choose. We need to be mindful that we can have control to make healthy choices, learn to block, manage our stress and enjoy our lives.

Stress often comes from feeling as though we have been painted into a corner and that we have no control over the situation. If we take a minute, however, to really think about all the options we actually have, it will often reduce our stress and help us feel better. The key is to pay attention before life becomes so stressful and make choices that will keep us off of a stressful path.

All of us make dysfunctional choices. It is part of being a human being. That is how we learn. That is how we develop into the person we become.

Since there are not enough mental health professionals in the world and not enough money in the pockets of people who really need them, I wish there was more in our society to encourage people and help them find their way onto a healthy path and a productive lifestyle.

I'm grateful I got to raise my children when the world was a friendlier place. The amount of pressure, negativity and stress in the world is overwhelming so many. Nonetheless, we must remember that we have a choice about blocking the negatively and staying positive with our decision making. We can do this!

In summary:

We must stop giving up our power!
We have the power to block!!
We have the power to respond positively.

We always have options.

Honoring our path is a choice.

Choosing "which self?" is a choice.

We must believe in ourselves, forge a positive path, and make healthy choices to honor our journey.

We can do this!

+≍+

1. As you consider your personal choices, is there one you want to re-think, re-decide and change?

2. Is there something or someone you need to work on blocking in order to enjoy a more peaceful life?

3. Envision making a different choice as a means of honoring your personal path. Make a plan for how you might go about making it a reality.

Chapter Two

DERAILED BY DETOURS

"Two roads diverged in a wood,
and I took the one less traveled by,
and that has made all the difference.
(Robert Frost)

Whoever we are, wherever we are on our journey, we got there one choice at a time. Most of them we made ourselves! If we don't like where we are, we have the power to make different choices.

We come into the world with parents we didn't get to choose. Maybe we didn't even want to come at all, or maybe we will decide not to stay.

We didn't get to choose our country, our nationality, the values others taught us about how to see the world, our DNA--so many things that impact our journey and sense of self.

We have to decide who and what we want our life to be, given the hand we've been dealt and choose how to play it out. Time is passing quickly and we won't always have those choices. Life is about now, always now. It's all about timing.

We end up having to figure out what having a healthy journey even means and make our own decision about how or whether to pursue it. At some point we also need to decide to understand that there are many ways in which our paths can be sabotaged, both by ourselves and by others. This is a very complex process.

Honoring our journey is probably the hardest work any of us will ever do. It requires that we use our wide-angle lens and view life and ourselves as honestly as we possibly can. In fact, we may even have to ask for some help to make it happen. There are people who can help.

Typically, in the process of constructing our journey, we all encounter blockages. Sometimes we try to find a way to go around them. What we don't understand is that the path around is usually longer and more painful than what we hoped it would help us avoid. This is, in fact, where detours are created. This is often when a mental health person is asked to intervene and help people cope.

Detours are choices we create to help us avoid pain. Sometimes, however, they become more painful than the pain they were designed to help us avoid. Ask any opioid user, or heroin user or alcoholic? I've treated them all. Detours are fun, until they aren't! Sometimes we realize what we're doing, other times we simply don't care.

I'm reminded of the interview between Whitney Houston and Oprah Winfrey in which Whitney was asked how she felt about being given "the gift-- her voice, a national treasure," and why she had not sung in 7 years. She answered that she had all the money, houses, cars, drugs she wanted and that she didn't even think about having "the voice." This is a prime example of getting lost on a detour.

Everyone creates detours. Everyone wants to avoid pain and numb out. Get in line!

Fear is often a major factor for creating detours--fear of rejection, fear of unknown consequences, fear of not being liked, fear of moving out of our comfort zone, and fear of failure. Parents often model these fears and pass them along to their children.

Detours can be deadly. There were more heroin overdoses in 2015 than deaths due to guns in the USA. We have a serious problem people.

Some people seek out detours, build a house on them, and die there. Often they bear children there who never get to see a healthy model of an honored journey. This makes it difficult for them to even understand what a healthy and honored journey would look like, let alone know how to go about having one. People's reality is built on their experiences. Be careful where you build.

Detours often have their foundations in such things as depression, addictions, insecurity, mental illness, alcohol, drugs, poverty, anger and can be precipitated by most anything. Often, we are a long way down the detour before we figure out what has happened, namely that we have turned whatever took us there and made it a lifestyle.

Nonetheless, we count on it to help us numb the pain. Once we cross those lines, we are starting the process of a habit which we may not be able to break. We must own the reality of the price we are paying for the time we spend on the detour. We will never get it back. What is the price tag attached to the detour(s)? Can we afford it?

I am reminded of a story of a man, a good man who made a bad choice, who chose a detour by marrying a woman he didn't love. After 10 years of marriage, when he had achieved his significant goal, he decided to disclose to her that he didn't love her, since he didn't need her anymore. Yet, she had made a critical decision to marry him, based on a lie. Now, ten years and 3 children later, she needed to choose how to handle this information, in the middle of feeling absolutely devastated.

What were her options? She could spend the rest of her life hating him, divorce him and try not to look back. Or, she could figure out a way to end the relationship rationally and look for ways to salvage what she could of her life, support her children, and move on. This is an example of the kinds of crises that happen every day. People face these kinds of heartbreaking crises every day around the world. Trauma is everywhere. It doesn't feel fair. It isn't fair. Nonetheless, it is a reality.

No wonder people get caught up in revenge, homicide and suicide. It is a crazy world in which we live. It is little wonder that people are so guarded, angry, hopeless, addicted, and full of rage and depression. What they need is to feel empowered in order to make healthy changes.

Since there are no perfect people, marriages or family, we soon figure out that honoring our journey is not so easy.

Then there is the issue of "rules." They are everywhere, written and unwritten. We first learn about them in our family system--the do's and don'ts of our family. We learn that when we cross over lines, we get punished. Then we go to school and learn about self-esteem and discover that acquiring some can be a daunting task. We find that we are constantly compared to others in a world that is often less than kind, where bullying and sexting have become the new normal. In the midst of all this mess, we are supposed to figure out how to have and maintain a positive sense of self. Good luck with that.

It is very difficult to create a path whereby we honor our journey when we don't really care about the person on the journey. Otherwise, we just get caught up in the crowds of life and go through the motions to make it to the end of the day and to the end of our lives.

I wrote both my Master's thesis and Ph.D. dissertation on the subject of self-esteem and wish I could report something positive about it. I have found few things as difficult as helping people believe in themselves.

Yet, without this foundation, life becomes very difficult to maintain, let alone honor. Statistics back up this fact since I learned that last year there were more deaths due to suicide in America than traffic fatalities. This is tragic.

What has gone so wrong in our society? In our parenting? In our schools? In our homes? In our hearts? In our values?

There are not enough mental health professionals or mental health funding to meet the needs of humanity. Our prisons are bursting and it would appear there is little rehabilitation going on. People are losing hope. Taking anti-depressant and pain killing drugs has become a multi-billion dollar industry. This is the detour of numbing out. Thousands each year are dying as a result. They have given up. Some of them were my friends.

It is clear that there is much to pull us off our goal of honoring our journey. There are detours everywhere. They can be fun. They are tempting.

They make us feel good (for a time) but most of them, in the end, are deadly and we cannot afford to choose them.

What is the answer? The answer lies in focusing on our choices. That is where our power lies. The good news is that if we don't like our life, then we can make different choices and get off the detours. We may need to ask for help to do it. There are people who can and will help you if you ask.

For example, we can decide to stop reinforcing the detour of fear, of avoiding risks, of working on our self-esteem, stop being afraid, meet life head-on and honor our journey. We can set goals, put foundations under them and find our way back to the healthy path by taking back our personal power. We can do this if we want it badly enough to pay the price to make it happen. This includes letting go of our addictions. As one addicted patient put it, "After my first hit of crack cocaine, I knew I would crawl through the sewers and beg for it." We should never underestimate the power of drugs to impact our lives.

We need a clear focus, a clearly spelled out change we can follow to put us where we need to go. We can hold our feet to the path and take responsibility for our choices. We can thrive!-- not simply survive.

All of us need a teachable spirit, no matter how much we think we already know. We must be open to change, to try new ways to approach our problems, even when we're terrified of moving out of our comfort zone.

Speaking of comfort zones, I have moved completely out of mine in order to write this book. I am taking this topic very seriously. I'm devoting a year of my life to writing this book. I have moved to a new State, with my clothes and my dog and am camped out at a desert facility to take on this challenge. I'm dealing each day with goals and detours that pull me off the path. I'm finding this challenge very difficult, but doable.

I have put myself in 'time out.' I'm in a State where I've never lived and where I know no one, in order to complete this project. I can tell you, with honestly, that I've been here for a short time and am already finding this to be a daunting task.

I'm actually putting myself to the test but feel as though I am being led and learning as I proceed down this unknown path. I am journaling daily to keep track of my feelings, thoughts and behavior. I'm understanding why this is the 'road less travelled.'

My goal is change. I keep a very detailed journal to keep track of myself. I have set goals and each day I am faced with the challenge of accountability in an attempt to become centered, grounded and focused.

I've also identified detours I use which keep me from my goals. They are in my face and I don't like it. Nonetheless, I'm dealing with them and seeking to learn from them. In spite of my love for learning, some days, I think I'd rather just have a root canal.

People in the field of mental health often struggle as hard as those they are treating. I am reminded of a horrible Easter Sunday I spent calling all of the patients of one of my psychologist colleagues who killed himself. I remember having to hold the phone far away from me as I listened to their sobs and screams of agony. Clearly, knowing isn't doing. Even psychologists end their lives.

Challenges come with our choices as well as how we respond to them. That is a key point. Everyone makes their own choices about how they choose to respond. Clearly, not everyone reaches the same conclusion. This has everything to do with the filter they are wearing, a filter based on their unique set of experiences.

We each manage stress in our own way. I make it a point to include monthly or weekly massages. They help me relax. Many adults simply don't care about themselves and do not make provisions for self-care. I've heard it said that our body is our auto-biography. How people care, or fail to take care, of themselves is communicated, in part, by their appearance.

I've heard it said that we are the carpenters of our own crosses. While this is not an especially popular belief, I think there is truth to the concept.

If we don't like our life, we need to make different choices. Usually, there is no one else to do it for us. The catch with making choices is that we must take responsibility for the outcome, regardless of what they are, and find a way to manage them. Blaming others is not the answer (even when they deserve to share the blame!) We don't save ourselves by destroying others.

Yesterday, I took time to look through my "friends' on my Facebook page and thought long and hard about whether or not we were friends. I deleted many of them. This was a painful reality for me, but better than kidding myself.

I don't think it matters how much money we have, the beauty of our physical appearance, how big our house or the make of car we drive. In the end, it's about our journey and how we feel about it. This becomes more apparent as we get closer to the end of our time. The goal is to let go with more peace than regrets, to feel good about what we did with what we were given. To whom much is given, much is required.

Think with me about the path. We all have a starting point but we have no idea where, when, or how it will end. The challenge, then, is to live each day as though it were our last.

I recently watched on T.V. the tragic story of the murder of the 6 year old, Jon Benet Ramsey, who died Christmas day in her home Boulder, Colorado, a mystery that is still unsolved 20 years later. I lived nearby at the time.

She had gotten a new bike for Christmas and was so excited. She and her Dad spent time helping her learn to ride it that day. She begged him for a few more minutes but he told her it was time to go, that they would do it "later." He said one of his great regrets is that he didn't take those few minutes to honor her request, because "later" will never come again for them. Life is now, and her little life was tragically ended unexpectedly.

We all need tools to help us honor our journey. We need help to navigate and make wise decisions to stay on track, even when it is rocky, barren, lonely and sometimes terrifying.

No matter what lies on the path, it is a better choice to face it than to create a detour to avoid it. It won't go away. We need strength of character to face it and continue to make healthy choices. We probably need to learn some tough love for ourselves.

I believe we need to learn to be our own best critic, and sometimes our own best friend. Somedays we need to create our own sunshine.

We need to take a hard, honest look at ourselves and determine if we need to make changes. If we do, we need to remember that a risk is a win. We are better off trying to make a change than die wondering how it might have changed our life if we had tried.

Detail and discipline are two of my least favorite tasks. Yet, I find them in my face every day as I make my way through this challenge. There has to be some joy and reinforcement of the goals in order to stay off the detours. I'm finding this easier said than done.

Eventually, this process of making healthy choices becomes reinforcing and very positive. We become stronger. Things become clearer. Our self-esteem increases and we feel gratified with our choices, as we take more pride in our healthy choice and our decision that got us there. However, we can't set a goal, then check on it in a year to see how we are doing. We have to set the goal, then put a foundation under it to reach it. We have to re-choose it every single day and make it a part of our path, something I call "chunking." That means that we set mini-goals to get us to where we want to be. It is actually a very powerful tool.

I can't say enough about raising our awareness of our choices. They are what is controlling our life. All of us face dozens of these challenges every day. The issue is what we do about them and whether or not we take responsibility for them. I believe we need to pay careful attention to which of the messages we are listening to inside our brain. We need to take control of that process.

As I indicated, a critical tool for success in life is having healthy self-esteem. It is hard not to allow the people around us to shape our life. We have to know and accept our strengths as well as our weaknesses and decide what really matters to us.

We can't expect people to accept, let alone praise us for our strengths which may only threaten them. We cannot expect them to respect our path if we don't. We also can't afford to let them direct our path if they do not have our best interests at heart. We all have to stop wanting people to be the way we want them to be in order to serve our own needs.

Also, we must control our boundaries. We must not violate our boundaries if we expect to maintain our positive self of self. I know this from personal experience. When we cross over lines we know are wrong and cross them anyway, we pay a price attached to that choice. It will cost us, sometimes for a lifetime. Many of these choices we cannot undo. That ship has sailed.

Another detour is in forming interpersonal relationships. Sometimes we want to be liked more than holding true to presenting ourselves genuinely. It is not wise to present ourselves as someone other than who we are. Remember, we have to like ourselves in order to make our life work. Otherwise, we present a façade of who we are and life begins to fall apart because we can't maintain it.

If others are intimidated by us and try to make us responsible for their feelings of inadequacy, they must take responsibility and not blame us for feeling "never good enough." That is what insecure people and bullies do. We must not give them that power. They have work to do on themselves! They must take responsibility for their own feelings, not blame it on others.

One of the pitfalls I sometimes fall into is that I turn people into who I want them to be and then get frustrated and disappointed when they don't turn out to be that person. Sometimes I get very blind-sighted and this becomes a painful reality. I'm working to change this pattern.

Throughout our lives, we will likely encounter people who will make it a point to rain on our parade, maybe even people in our own family. We must remember that the things people say about others always says more about them than the person they are describing.

It is very sad to me that children are unable to grasp this concept as I have witnessed the deadly effects of bullying when I dealt with the Columbine High School tragedy. It enrages me, to this day!! Today I read about a 5 year old boy who refused to get on the school bus because he was being bullied. The police found him walking alone on a highway. ENOUGH!!!

We need to develop the tool of affirming others, calling attention to their strengths, gifts and abilities but we can only do this if our own self-esteem is intact. We need to build each other up, not tear each other down. Everyone we meet needs positive reinforcement. Sometimes, we have to provide it for ourselves, be the sunshine we need in our lives.

Another helpful tool is to consider the price tag attached to our choices. When we choose a mate, have a child, take our first drink or street drug and pretend that none of this really affects who we are, then we need to ask ourselves a question: "What am I pretending not to know?"

As a psychologist, I have had to tilt my head back during sessions so the tears didn't run down my face, particularly during the five years I worked with severely abused and traumatized children who had been removed from their homes by the Courts. I've had to close files I was reading about inmate patient crimes for fear of vomiting. I've had to close my note pad during a session where I'm being told what it's like to rape a four year old. I've had my life threatened more than once by mentally ill inmates. I watched a man electrocute himself six feet in front of me. I've left the maximum security prison parking lot, after a ten hour work day, thinking, "I hate everyone."

I've used up a lot of my defenses, something I didn't discover until long after I stopped doing that work. I have discovered the reality of the price I paid to get involved with being a mental health professional, something I never remember being discussed during graduate school.

Personally, I have come to the realization, since retiring, of the significance of my choice to pursue mental health in various settings. I feel privileged to have done the work I did. I do not regret it but am acutely aware of the impact it has had on me. The point I am making is that there are very real consequences attached to our choices and we would all do well to be aware of this fact.

When I think about my own efforts to deal with detours, I am reminded of a very personal truth. Someone died who hurt me more deeply than I could imagine. Since one of my detours is anger/ rage, I grasped the urgency of my need to deal with this event. I played a song that represented all of the good feelings I used to have about this person. I forced myself to listen to the entire song, with my head in my hands, sobbing, forcing myself to remember all of the incredibly positive feelings I once had for this person. Painfully, I stayed with it until I could honestly express my feelings of "rest in peace" and mean it. What an enormous challenge for me to do what I needed to do in order to stay off the detour of anger and bitterness. I'm very grateful I could do it. Thankfully, those angry feelings have not returned.

In truth, the challenge of deciding what we want our journey to be, figuring out ways to honor our choices, and deciding every single day to be our best, is an enormous challenge for us all.

So, where does it all really begin? I believe a key tool for all of us is to fully accept the hand we have been dealt--the positives and the negatives--and get really honest about how we choose to play it out. This is where it all really begins.....and ends.

One thing is certain: the detours are deadly.

1. Identify the detours you use and identify what you are trying to avoid.

2. Contemplate a plan for change for each of your detours, by chunking them out.

3. Set some new fun and personal goals for yourself, things you really enjoy, things that will help you avoid the need for detours.

Chapter Three

LEARNING TO REFRAME

"Life is what happens to us while
we're busy making other plans."

Learning to reframe our experiences is, I believe, a very valuable tool to have in our life skills toolbox. It is the ability to understand an event from an entirely different point of view. It is like taking a picture and putting it in a different frame.

For example, the pain of divorce can be excruciating, especially for children. However, they can learn that they have two good parents who love them very much and their lives will go on, not as before, but they will always be loved by and love their parents. They come to understand that not everyone can spend their lives together, even if they love each other. People are sometimes simply not compatible with one another. This is a reframe.

No matter who we are, or where we are, in our efforts at honoring our journey, we need to understand that everyone has a different exam, that is, we each have our own unique personal space, value system and set of challenges. It is different for each of us. We must respect our own journey, no matter what the circumstances, and stop judging others.

All of us undergo many changes in our lives which send us down paths we never would have believed or chosen. There is so much of it over which we have no control. All we can control are our responses. This is a profound reality where reframing can serve us well.

Speaking for myself, I would never have envisioned my life to be what it has become. If my many decades of marriage had not ended, I would never have done any work with abused children or violent offenders. If I hadn't had my work place accident, I would never have written any books. I have had to constantly reframe my life in order to determine the direction. There were always choices, but it was up to me to decide what the reframe would be and how I would go about working to fulfill it. To put it mildly, I have found this to be an amazing challenge. I remember thinking, "Well....if I'm no longer a wife......and no longer a mother on a daily basis.....and

I'm no longer an employed psychologist, then who am I?

I learned through this experience that each of us has to come to terms with the unique circumstances that may occur in our lives. So much of life just seems to be out of our control, no matter how we might envision it. When that happens, we need to find a way to reframe our circumstances. That is, we need to find a way to reframe and move forward, easy to say, hard to do!

I believe part of the teachable spirit is to understand and accept that things will happen to us that really are out of our control and they will change the trajectory of our lives, fair or unfair. We don't always get to choose how things will turn out.

We are not the only player on our path, and most of us do not see what is in our future. Others can wreak havoc with us in a million ways. We must stay teachable, be able to reframe, and be determined to continue moving forward, no matter what. Giving up should never be considered an option!

No matter what we believe, our challenge is to discern and make the wisest choices we can. In playing out our hand, we need to discern the best choices we can, then make adjustments as required, and keep moving forward. We reframe in order to stay positive and not create a detour. This thing called life is complex and very difficult, even under the best of circumstances. Everyone walks with a limp of some kind. It is extremely challenging even for those of us who have acquired advanced degrees in the managing of it. Knowing isn't doing!!

I have met people who have suffered unbelievable things, yet they can find a way to reframe and move on. I have also met people who have suffered a little and their mantra has become, "Ain't it awful." While this seems to me to be a real waste of time, I have tried hard to work with and be patient with those people. During my private practice, I listened to various versions of this theme for several months from several different people.

However, at some point I intervened by raising the issue of exploring the possibility of using their good energy toward seeking productive solutions to problems. As long as we are focused on our hurt feelings (even justified ones) of the wrongs others have done to us, if our life becomes about those people and their behaviors, they are still controlling us. We are allowing them to continue to hurt us. Those behaviors require being redirected so they can be worked through, put on a shelf and move forward. We need to learn to let go--something very hard to do. Nonetheless, I know it is possible. I have lived it. Reframing is essential to mental health.

In my own life, when I have felt stuck, I have sought out the few I know whom I believe would be honest me, not tell me what they thought I wanted to hear. The way we learn and grow is to be brutally honest with ourselves about the ways we are thinking and the choices we are making. Only a very good friend (far too few of those) will be honest with us and speak the truth in love so we can hear and accept it. I believe it is one of the greatest human acts of love we can show each other. They can help us find a better path. Sometimes we just have to reach out and ask for help. We need to train ourselves to pay attention to our own inner dialogue and learn to let it go when angry, bitter thoughts take over.

I have found that I use the phrase to myself every single day: "Let it go!" In fact, I use it more than ever, as my awareness has increased. I'm learning to let go of what I'm not able to reframe. Actually, sometimes the letting go IS the reframe!!

It isn't easy for anyone to have to hear they are using up their good energy in non-productive ways, that there is a much better way. In fact, the anger we intend to be directed towards others usually ends up hurting us more than anyone. They are not worth all of that angst. We must stop blaming all of the people in our lives (who may even deserve blame) and determine not to allow them to hurt us anymore. We can't afford to go there. Hanging onto it hurts us, not them. We must find a way to reframe it and move forward.

Many of us have traumatic childhood memories. They were totally unfair and scarred us deeply. But, when we become adults, we have the choice to reframe our pain and keep moving forward, determined to honor our journey. I know this is possible. I've lived it.

My childhood was one of the most painful periods of my life. It took me many years to learn, and unlearn, with professional help, how to do what I'm talking about here. Hanging onto painful memories translates to baggage we can't afford to carry. It is, however, a decision each person must decide for themselves. Others can help us understand what we're doing, but, ultimately, each of us must make the decision we can live with.

Our path is rarely straight. It weaves and careens near the precipice on many parts of our journey. It is often painful and challenging, sometimes taking us to a breaking point. Letting go of all that pain is a process, not an event. It happens slowly, as we release little pieces of our pain, a day at a time.

I have taught the course of Anger Management in many settings. My own experience has taught me that I have to go through my feelings of anger and rage and own them before I can let go of them. An exercise I sometimes use is to imagine that person is sitting in a chair and I express what I'm feeling about them. I actually talk to them out loud. I have to go through the ashes to emerge to a better space. In fact, I recall once when I was in therapy, expressing the thought, "I hate you so much, I can't find enough hate to hate you with." Clearly, I had work to do.

Therapy is rarely a quick fix and will probably always be unfinished business. Yet, in my many years of private practice I often found that the last question of the first session would be, "How long is this going to take?" to which I would reply, "How long did it take you to get like this?"

Many people are looking for a quick fix. Yet I know of no one with any magic who can provide it. In fact, I looked long and hard for it myself rather than do all the work I knew I had in front of me. There is no magic and no quick fixes. That is what we call 'magical thinking.'

I am a strong believer in the concept of forgiveness but I don't believe it happens quickly or easily. I believe it is a process whereby we give up little pieces of our pain over time which eventually leads us to a better place. It requires commitment and determination. It is very hard work and often re-emerges only to have to be dealt with again and again. Those are the moments when I repeat to myself, "....just let it go....." This helps.

As part of my Ph.D. in Clinical Psychology, I was required to accrue 40 hours of therapy as a patient with a board certified psychiatrist or psychologist. I chose a psychiatrist, board certified from Harvard. I learned many things from him, mostly what it felt like to be so vulnerable in sharing my closely-guarded painful secrets. To this day, I often think of what I learned there and how it continues to help me in honoring my journey. My doctor passed away a few years but he left me a cherished legacy for my life toolbox. I will be forever grateful, though the process did not always feel good. I know what it's like to spend your life telling people things they probably don't want to hear.

Without a teachable spirit, we are likely going to experience a very long, painful and lonely life. We must make the choice to learn to stay open to new ideas. There is so much we can learn from one another if we will just take the time and make the effort to simply listen to each other and to our heart as well.

One of the ways I work to stay grounded and focused is to set goals, then work to put a foundation under them and hold myself accountable as I work on them. During this process, I discover whether or not I am really committed to my goal or whether it is simply something I think would be nice but find that I am not willing to do the work required to reach the goal. This is a learning process, sometimes a painful one. Clearly, it is a way of keeping track of who we are and what we really want. It helps to clarify our path. It is often two steps forward, three steps back.

Our actions tell the tale. If we say we want something, but our behavior tells us otherwise, then we need to get honest with ourselves and own it. This is one of the reasons I journal my thoughts, feelings and behavior. It is a way of keeping track of myself. It seems the more I learn, the more I realize how much I still need to learn, and how little I know.

When my children were grown, I was no longer married or employed, it posed a real challenge to me as to what my life would become. Pain is a powerful motivator. I found the challenge not to be what I wanted to DO but rather who I wanted to BE, what I wanted my life to be about. I thought about what I wanted to be able to feel about my life when it was over. It motivated me to work on my unfinished business.

I am now months into my new "time out" venture earlier described. I continue to challenge myself and hold myself accountable. I am also learning how difficult it is to set a goal and stay committed to it.

I cannot emphasize enough how critical our internal dialogue is and the choices we make about which of them we are going to choose to listen to and act on. I am learning to develop internal messages that say, "Yes, I can!" and "No, I won't!"

I'm learning about myself and the process of change. I'm learning that discipline and consistency are difficult. I'm learning that I can't do it perfectly. I'm learning that some days I don't feel like doing it at all. I'm doing better in some areas than others. I've had some very discouraging days.

I'm succeeding better in some areas than others but, no matter what, I am learning and making continuous adjustment based on that learning. I am concentrating on putting one foot in front of the other and trusting the ground to be there.

Learning is not always a 'feel good' experience. Some new pieces of information cause us pain and discouragement. However, this is usually where real learning begins. If we can learn from our mistakes and allow them to guide us in a different direction, then we are reframing and learning from them. This is good. The trick is not to do it perfectly. The trick is to simply do it!

A few months ago, I stopped taking a certain medication because I didn't like the way it made me feel. However, when I met a new internist, he explained to me in no uncertain terms that I really needed to take it. Once again I started taking it. I'm learning (reframing) that I can't structure my life simply based on what is comfortable for me. I must make wise decisions based on what is right for me to do. I'm learning that, instead of being resentful toward people who help me see I am making poor choices, I need to be open to hearing them and making changes. This is not an easy lesson to learn. Once again, knowing isn't doing!

If everyone could learn and apply the tool of reframing, we could mostly do away with a lot of rage and a lot of depression. Re-framing enables us to manage our lives in healthy ways, to make the necessary changes needed to honor our journey. It empowers us to make life adjustments as they are needed. It enables us not to carry baggage which only weighs us down.

In the end, it really isn't so much about what happens to us that determines our journey, is our ability to reframe and hold firm to our awareness that we have a choice about how we are going to respond. In the end, life seems to have a way of making us all accountable, whether we want to be or not. Karma is alive and well.

We need to protect ourselves by not watering the seeds of bitterness in our heart or allow vengeance to guide our life. That is a path from which we may never recover.

We need to make reframing our friend. It will help us honor our journey. We need to include it in our toolbox of mental health and use it often.

Practice it. Live it. It will change your life.

1. Identify an event in your life you need to reframe. How might you go about it?

2. What, specifically, do you need to reframe in order to honor your journey?

3. Think of the relief you can bring to yourself and others by making the effort to reframe what you need to, and can. Make it happen.

Chapter Four

RISKING CHANGE

"A risk is a win."

Part of mental health is having the ability to block and to remember that people's opinions about us really says more about them than about us. Unfortunately, this is a reality usually learned late in life, if at all.

We must use our tools and not allow others (or even ourselves) to send us into depression and fear, to destroy our lives. Many respond by creating detours. Many never find their way back to the path of the person they once believed they could be.

People lose hope and many of them simply give up. I have met far too many of these people. They have given up their lives for people they counted on to love them.....and didn't.

I still remember administering a sentence-completion test to little children with an item that read "Nobody cares......" Their response would almost always be "about me." This was heartbreaking.

I can recount many sessions with children who had experienced a family suicide. These people will never completely heal. Children who discover dead parents, parents who discover dead children--this kind of anguish doesn't go away. These are stories of trauma from which many never recover. I've heard far too many of these encounters. I recall a teenager who adored her Dad, who remembers him tucking her in bed one night when she was 4 years old who then went to the front yard and hanged himself!

Experiences change people. The power family members have over one another is hard to comprehend. In the 21st century, there appears to be so many reports in the media over family members who attack and kill one another. Statistics tell us we are more likely to be killed by someone we know, maybe even someone in our own family.

That was, of course, before we heard of ISIS which might behead you, set you on fire, make you a sex slave or drown you in an iron cage. What has happened to our world? These are barbaric acts people are clamoring to join. This is scary! It reminds me of psychological experiments that had to be terminated because of human brutality. These are terrifying times in our society.

What has happened to the concept of the family as the resource for providing a loving support system where we find acceptance, strength, comfort and support? It's more like, "If only I could relate to the people I'm related to."

The challenge of change is enormous, even when it's something we really want to change. If only it were that easy. If only someone really did have some magic or pill to make the change. It simply doesn't happen that way. We get hurt, we grieve, we get angry, we get depressed, we get even, but we don't get over it. Ultimately, we have to decide how much power we are going to give it to impact our journey.

Change is one of the most difficult challenges. I'm experiencing this daily, and I'm working hard at it. I believe it takes enormous commitment every single day. It means living outside of our comfort zone. Often it means giving up one of our major detours for coping with life. It is far easier to settle for the "crappy, but familiar" lifestyle we have adopted. We hate it, but it has become predictable. People usually do not want to move out of their comfort zone and work on changing. It is just too much work for them to choose it.

This is why it is so important to put healthy habits in place at an early age. If we are fortunate enough to grow up in a healthy family system, this is possible. However, most of us do not. These unhealthy habits often get passed from one generation to the next, and so it goes.... on and on......

Our free will allows us to be anyone we choose. At the same time, we begin to learn lessons about rules and consequences.

I believe we all adhere to some kind of internal value system which we have bought into that drives our behavior. After a while, it is so much a part of us that it doesn't even occur to us that we have the option to choose differently.

It's been said that most of us are the carpenters of our own crosses and that we can't un-ring the bell. Nonetheless, the possibility of change is, in fact, reality. I believe in it. I've seen it. It IS possible. However, getting people to believe it is the hard part. To many, this just sounds like a fairy tale.

My experience of people who seek our professional help with personal problems seldom includes their wanting to change. It is often to seek out validation for themselves of their negative feelings about the wrongs others have done to them. They are wanting to justify their revenge. They want to be comforted. They want to hear that they are "right." I sometimes ask them if they would rather be 'right' or well.?'

Somehow, it seems to offend people when it is suggested they might do an assessment of their own behaviors and see how they contributed to their problems or how they could change their lives for the better. Conflicts usually include at least two different points of view. There is usually some learning for all of us when we consider this fact. This is not a popular intervention.

It is my opinion that most of us give others far too much power to affect us, causing us to feel negatively about ourselves. If someone betrays us or turns out to not be our friend, we become hurt or angry, then we often self-sabotage, "What's the matter with me?" We go through a litany of options: "I'm not smart enough; I'm not pretty enough; I'm not rich enough; I'm not thin enough." We look for all of our faults, all the ways in which we already feel inadequate, and we sometimes just give up altogether. I've seen it happen. The other option is to unleash our rage on the person who has hurt us. Unfortunately, this often includes children and animals. I hate the evil perpetrated on the innocents.

I really believe many people carry around a sizeable chunk of themselves labelled, "Never good enough" which keeps us from all kinds of good things. Usually, we blame others for these feelings.

We need to understand that others cannot make us feel a certain way about ourselves unless we cooperate with them. I once heard a woman say to another, "You have just about destroyed me., to which the person replied, "Don't give me that much power."

Belittling, bullying, bribing, demanding change simply doesn't work. Nurturing, building up, reinforcing another person's gifts, offering praise, these are the building blocks of change. We need to give them to others and to ourselves.

It has been said, "I am not who I think I am. I am not who you think I am. I am who I think that you think that I am." This simply refers to how people conclude who they are. I recently read of an abandoned 4 year old child who was asked her name. She replied, "Stupid....my name is stupid."

This says it all. How totally pathetic!

It has been my experience that low self-esteem people can be extremely critical in their judgment of others. The only way they can feel good about themselves is to bring others down as low as they feel about themselves. They can actually become very dangerous people.

Oftentimes, we end up wanting things from these people who simply don't have it to give to us. This includes children who need nurturance from a parent who doesn't have it to give. This is a very difficult interpersonal issue to treat. It is also a very painful reality to accept. Not everyone knows how to love.

Sometimes people try to change for someone else. Clearly, this does not work. We have to make the choice to change because it is our choice, not so someone will like us better. The real question is what do we need to change in order to like ourselves better?!

We need to develop a worldview that we believe in, that represents who we are, develop a filter we respect and believe in and use it to make any changes we choose. There are big prices to pay if we don't (and if we do!).

At the end of the day, as we look in the mirror, that person is the one we need to like and believe in. That is the one whose truth we need to practice. Our truth needs to matter to us, regardless of how others feel about it.

We must care more about what we think of ourselves than what other people think of us. The speaking of our truth is a reflection of who we are. This is foundational to honoring our journey.

The late social worker, Virginia Satir, once wrote that only 4 1/2% of the population engage in what she called "levelling" communication. This is communication that speaks our truth. Wouldn't the world be a much healthier place if we could count on people to actually do this? People are, unfortunately, dishonest because of feared consequences, mostly of not being liked.

I grew up in a very angry family. There was never any doubt how anyone felt about anything. This environment depressed me. Unknowingly, I picked up a lot of that style of communicating as a child because I thought that is how all families related. I remember a seventh grade teacher who wrote on my report card, "Needs to learn tact." I'm certain she was right.

It has taken me a long time to not be afraid of the expression of anger, but I have come to appreciate how high the bar was set in my family of origin for hostility.

I have worked for decades on trying to find the balance. My first Ph.D. is in Interpersonal Communications. I have worked very hard to become comfortable with my truth and try to always remember to speak it appropriately. Actually, I admire and respect people I perceive as authentic. I tend to trust them.

I am now well along in my personal time-out challenge. It is tedious, detailed, demands discipline and I sometimes feel a lot of resistance to it.

I continue to camp out in the desert with my card table, laptop, printer, clothes and my dog. Sometimes I feel challenged about the wisdom of choosing this project. Nonetheless, the dye has been cast and I am determined to complete the commitment.

I remember the days when I lived in a nearly 4,000 square foot 3 story home of oak and glass, on two acres, brand new. I am learning to respect that was my life then, this is my life now. There is so much to be learned, no matter where we are, or who we are. No matter what, we must accept our circumstances and find a way to live with and make the best of them.

I encourage you to examine the dynamics of your own life, take a hard look at the core of you and ask yourself if there are any changes you need to make. Start with a simple goal, chunk it out, reach it, then tackle another one. This is how progress is made.

Be all you can be. Commit to making any changes you need to in order to get you there. Contemplate, if your life was to end today, what change would you most regret not making?

I have spent a fair amount of time talking with people about their greatest regrets. We must all own the fact that our time will run out for making changes. We need to do what we can while we can.

Pay attention to the core of you. Do what you can while you can. Follow your heart. Timing is everything. Many of us find it difficult to even take the time to assess what we need to be doing. We are simply too busy trying to do 'life.'

The best and wisest things you and I can do for the people we love is to take care of ourselves. If we are fully functioning people, we will be much more likely to be a good role model and treat the people around us with respect and integrity, especially those who live under our own roof.

You and I get one chance, one life. This is not a dress rehearsal and we must not treat it like one if we expect to come to the end of it with many feelings of satisfaction. We must stop thinking we have forever to make changes. We don't.

I am aware of recent tragedies around the world whereby loved one's lives have ended forever. Recently, six elementary school children died when their school bus crashed. Dozens of Christmas shoppers have been run down by terrorists as they went about their lives. When will it happen to one of our loved ones?

To ourselves? We never think it will be us. We're wrong.

We have all had experiences we wish we could change. We can't. I will never forget watching my oldest son pitch the ball to a young teenager who hit the ball, made it to third base and dropped dead. And, I remember driving home late one night, coming over a hill and saw a body lying in the middle of the road as the result of an accident which had just happened. There is daily trauma going on around the world. We are all affected.

We need to learn from traumatic events, ours and others, and make changes while we still can. Some of the simple changes I have made include: going into a store at Christmas time where parents are buying toys for their children, find someone who is needy and help them by buying toys and providing Christmas dinner. I give monthly to help abused animals. When I cross a major bridge, I pay for myself and for the car behind me. These are just little things but they represent paying it forward. It is a way of being congruent since I believe I am my brother's keeper.

If everyone did little things to pay it forward, it would be life changing in the world. Our behaviors should reflect our values.

Life is NOW. We need to be realistic in assessing where we are in our life currently. If we are living a lie, living someone else's life, living miserably, then it's time to be thinking about making changes. I think we also need to be thinking about how our choices impact the people around us. What do they need for us to change? Making changes is a risk. Life is a risk. Relationships are a risk. We need to get honest about it all and get serious about making changes.

I once lived with a good friend during the last year of her life. She had terminal cancer. She was 45 years old, a single parent with 3 children. I learned so much from her through her dark days of pain and struggle. What a privilege it was to spend those days with her. I was with her when she took her last breath, closed her eyes and accepted the reality and finality of her death.

I don't think I could ever do that for anyone again. Death was in my face and I'll never forget it. Letting in and letting go is some of the hardest work humans must do.

People pass in and out of our lives as we pass through theirs. We need to fully embrace them while we have that incredible opportunity so that when it comes time to let them go, we can do it, without regret and with peace and cherished memories.

This is an important and difficult reality to grasp.

1. Identify a change you know you need to make.

2. Take time to plan out a strategy for making the change.

3. Make your life more enjoyable and make the change to do something each day that nurtures yourself.

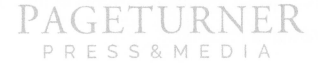

Chapter Five

SHOWING COMPASSION

"....the greatest of these is love..."

The movie star Edward Norton recently made a statement at a televised CNN event that "Helping others is far sexier than any movie star." How great that someone from Hollywood would praise acts of kindness in contrast to the Hollywood fixation on sex. I found this refreshing and encouraging.

I once conducted a research study at a university where I was teaching a course on Interpersonal Communications. I took a survey, asking what was the most important personal quality of a person most valued by others. Ironically, the answer wasn't beauty, sexy, talent, intelligence or wealth. It was compassion! Who knew?

Compassion means we care. Compassion means we will take the time to listen. Compassion means putting aside our own needs to help others. Compassion means we go the second mile. Compassion means we give a damn! Compassion is part of a value system.

Compassion means we seek to know what love even looks like to those we care about and want to express it. Where are those people? Where did those beautiful faces go?

Compassion is a quality we can work to integrate into our lifestyle. It is like having a personal mission statement that wants to make a difference for good, one that has a basic caring attitude toward all people.

I don't believe I have ever witnessed a period during my lifetime with less compassion. Man's inhumanity to man is a new normal that I abhor. Every day, we read in the media about death of children from road rage, torture of children and animals, soaring drug and homicide rates, gang violence, sex trafficking of children, etc. Whatever became of compassion? When did we stop being our brother's keeper? When did others' pain no longer concern us? What has happened to our society that we no longer seem to care? and take the attitude, "It's not my problem." Instead, our focus is on greed, on ourselves, on "What's in it for me?"

I guess I'm still 'old school.' I remember the days when neighbors mattered, when we took the time to try to be respectful of and honoring to others, when a handshake meant something. I remember when surrounding neighbors took food or baked goods to a new neighbor who moved into their neighborhood, to welcome them. I remember when people counted on each other, where people helped because they wanted to, not so it would result in some kind of personal gain.

Somehow, it seems harder in today's world to trust the motives of others. Compassion still exists but it seems far less evident. People are hungry for compassion and finding it seems difficult. It doesn't appear to be a very big part of the new normal. The new normal seems to depersonalize people. I believe it hurts people. We receive depersonalized Christmas cards, if at all, ...and Christmas, it appears, is one of the saddest days of the year for many.... a big reminder of all that isn't in the world and isn't in their lives.

The new normal seems to be a society which glorifies violence! Bullying and sexting have become barbaric art forms. We are paying an enormous price for it in our lives and in our families, not to mention our physical and mental health.

The human spirit needs to know that it can count on others, that there are those who really do care. I've never seen man's inhumanity to man at this level. Where are we headed? Our foster children's placements are at an all-time high. Children need to be loved and need healthy role models to help them find their way to honoring their journey. It isn't happening!

I admit that I have spent a large portion of my life, trafficking at the seamy end of society and it has, no doubt, raised my awareness of negativity and mental illness. This week, I was made aware that a child I treated at age 7 was just arrested recently for strangling to death a pregnant woman. I can't begin to describe my feelings.

I have actually looked into the eyes of evil on more than one occasion and I'll never forget it. I've stood on death row at a major prison and felt the overwhelming negative energy that felt like a tidal wave from hell. I have experienced the reality of the impact of mental illness as well as evil. It is hellacious.

I am well trained in the arena of mental illness, but not in the treatment of evil. There is a decided difference. Many mentally ill and evil people are without a conscience. They experience no remorse for their behaviors. They love things and use people, not the other way around. I find them to be very dangerous people. We are wise to be wary of them.

In recent years, after my experience on death row, I changed my attitude regarding capital punishment. I am now in favor of it, whereas I never was before. After witnessing the impact of evil upon the innocents, I must honestly admit it enrages me. I have treated young children who are insane due to physical, sexual and emotional trauma. I cannot even find the words to describe my feelings.

I recall in the movie, "On Golden Pond" the famous line where Katherine Hepburn says, "Sometimes you just have to look at a person and realize they are doing the best they can." This is a compassionate approach to human beings, one we would all do well to apply to those around us, especially those under our own roof.

Everyone needs compassion. We need to gift it to ourselves as well. No one is perfect, we all make mistakes, but creating a detour of hate and vengeance is not the answer! We are a planet of angry people who act out in all kinds of ways. We need to turn this around. It will take all of us to make a difference.

One of the evidences of compassion is when we pay it forward, when we go out of our way to try to make a positive difference for someone. We can make some kind of donation to the volunteer ringing the bell at Christmas time, we can volunteer some of our time and money for people and animals who desperately need it. We can care, and do something to show it.

It doesn't always turn out the way we hoped, but at least we know we tried. We can only be accountable for our behavior, not the response.

We never know when it could be us who needs help. None of us are above losing our jobs, getting sick, losing loved ones, contemplating suicide, sleeping under the bridge, etc. The day may come when we are the ones who may need for someone to pay it forward and help us. We would do well to stay reminded of this fact.

Empathy begins when we are able to imagine ourselves in the hurting person's life and realize how we might feel if we were that person. Truth be told, none of us really know the path that others are walking and the challenges they are facing. We all need compassion.

What I am really getting at here is our awareness of our own internal dialogue. We constantly screen internal thoughts and decide which ones to act on. This is the nature of human beings interacting and communicating. We need to pay attention to and filter our responses. The messages we send to others has everything to do with how we think they will respond to us.

I think the goal is to speak our truth 'in love,' whatever it may be.

People notice how they feel in our presence. While we are not responsible for their feelings, we do need to be aware of the messages we are sending, positive and negative. People seek affirmation. People deserve compassion.

What about 'self-compassion?' Are we able to have empathy for ourselves? I've known many who struggle hard with self-forgiveness. We have trouble letting go of the mistakes we have made. Yet, we need to find a way to keep it from turning into excess baggage we can't afford to carry.

Most of seek out a compassionate other when we are hurting. Sometimes we can't find one. This makes life difficult. An example of this is the life of caretakers. They are one of the most depressed groups of people on the planet. They give and give and give until they feel given out. I'm thinking of those who have physically ill and mentally ill family members whom they feel compelled to help but that challenge feels overwhelming at times and creates anger and frustration. It costs to care!

Compassion is a choice, as is having a critical and judgmental attitude. It is easy to see shortcomings in others, and in ourselves. Sometimes we have to look harder to see the gifts, talents and struggles of that person, and offer an encouraging word. We also need to do it for ourselves. This is a very valuable tool to develop. It keeps us focused. It is a great tool for maintaining mental health. We need to maintain an inner attitude to do the best we can and let it be enough.

My own journey has taught me that I 'can't fix it.' I have learned to focus more on my own behaviors, less on others. All we can do is try our best, and learn from our mistakes. This is part of honoring our journey.

Do we know what compassion and love look like to the people in our family? If we do know, do we give love to them on their terms, not ours?

Life has taught me that what I want to give is sometimes not what people really need from me. I have learned to try to listen hard to what they are telling me and respond in kind. This is very hard to do if we are not honoring our own journey, and theirs!

I can still recall an incident decades ago when I spent Christmas eve with an unbeliever. Yet, he suggested we attend a Christmas eve service. I didn't appreciate the specialness of that gesture at the time nearly as much as I do now. He was showing me love on my terms. I didn't get it at the time. He was thinking of me, not himself. What a treasure he was. I'm sorry I never told him. Now, I'll never have that chance. Compassion and love make all the difference and sometimes we find it in unlikely places. In the end, I doubt any of us will regret the time we took to communicate compassionate and loving responses to others and to ourselves. We will likely cherish those memories, as will others.

Everyone needs positive reinforcement and nurturance. If we don't get it from others, then we need to provide it to ourselves. That is what keeps us on the path and off of the detours. We need to honor our needs and be compassionate with our weaknesses. In short, we need to stay focused and honor our journey. Some days we will need to create our own sunshine.

We need to dare to develop a psychological filter whereby we see ourselves and others through a compassionate lens. This can make a world of difference in the receiver's life as well as our own. Curb the critical spirit. Speak the truth in love. Treat others the way you want them to treat you. Be all you can be, every day of your life.

I can't help but think of Jesus' response to the woman who was caught in adultery. "Let him that is without sin cast the first stone." This says it all. It makes me wince to recount all the stones I have thrown and continue to feel the pain of those that have been thrown at me.

Compassion, I believe, needs to be a goal for all of us. It can change the world, and the people who choose to practice it.

Speaking frankly, I believe there is also a bit of a downside to compassion and that is having the expectation that it is going to have the hoped for outcome we desire. That doesn't always happen.

As I indicated earlier, a child I treated many years ago has been charged with committing murder and will likely spend the rest of her life incarcerated or executed. As it turns out, this was the only client in my entire career I ever felt fear of, even when she was a young child. I tried in every way I knew to help her. This is a sobering reminder to me that no matter who we are or how much we want good things for others, it is always up to them, not us, to make it happen.

It was a very disturbing reminder to me that even when we do show compassion to others, ultimately it is their decision to decide who they choose to be. We can only do our part. It is not a perfect world and there are at least a million different variable that affect outcomes. There are no guarantees, no matter what. What a hard lesson this has been for me to learn...

At the end of the day, as I reflect upon my actions, I ask myself whether or not I treated others the way I want to be treated. I don't always get the answer I hoped for. This is an opportunity to learn, assess and make changes. I must choose the actions I know I can live with and take responsibility for them. It is a constant learning and assessment process.

At the end of the day, what I remember most about compassion is:

"....the greatest of these is love...."

1. Identify an act of compassion that you could do that would help someone.

2. Identify a plan for accomplishing compassion.

3. Find a way that is comfortable for you to enjoy showing compassion to others.

Make it happen.

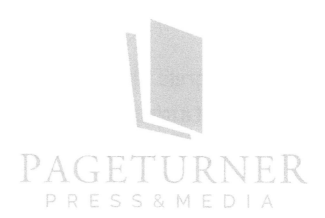

Chapter Six

MANAGING REGRETS

"I thought I grew, but here I am again..."

Everyone has regrets. The challenge appears to be to keep them at a minimum while increasing positive behaviors that make us proud to honor our journey.

Sometimes regrets are completely out of our control. It may be something done by someone else and we cannot undo their behavior. Rejection of all kinds fit this category. Families split apart, parent-child conflicts, road rage, international conflicts, so much that creates massive regrets and pain for so many. Life can be very unfair and many innocent people suffer great pain.

Then there exists the regrets that are in our control, things we wish we had done, or had never done. We can apologize but we can't take it back. The bell has rung; it is what it is. Regrets come in all shapes and sizes and can occur at any time. We all make mistakes. Perhaps the important part is to learn from them so we don't repeat those behaviors. However, I've met some people who have never recovered from them. They simply can't let go.

Sometimes their answer is to simply give up. This is tragic. I have attended more than one funeral of those who decided not to try anymore.

My point here is that regrets are a very complex issue that messes with our lives and our relationships, as well as our mental health. I have spoken with adults who feel as though their whole life has been regretful. Finding their way out of the maze of regret is not easy to do.

The secret appears to not do things we know we will regret. Regrets are very personal. Often, they become our secrets we share with no one. We may feel ashamed, terrified, or simply like a very bad person. Regrets can eat people alive. I've seen it.

I know I have recounted things in my own life I have done that I know I can never take back, but always wish that I could. Living with our regrets is like living with an extra hundred pounds of weight on our body. It makes all of life harder. It is extra baggage that makes life and honoring our journey much harder.

Let's face it, there are some things we cannot change. We have to accept the hand we were dealt, no matter what. So many people spend their lives being angry and resentful about the hand they were dealt. This anger can give way to vengeance which can end up being very dangerous to others. I have actually had to warn others during my private practice when I became personally aware of a physical threat to them. Warning them to a stated physical threat is the law in mental health.

Mental and physical illnesses are always regretful. Yet, we must find a way to manage the facts of our lives and find a way to live with them. We all have some kind of handicap, something we wish hadn't come our way. But, it did and rather than denying it, we need to find a way to accept it and continue on as best we can. We need to find a way to reframe it and move forward.

Our experiences change us. When someone rejects us, we regret the pain it causes us. They may even apologize, but it doesn't take away our pain. Everyone seems to hurt everyone if they interact long enough. It seems to be the shape of love. We do, indeed, hurt the ones we love. Sometimes they are the only ones we trust enough to be honest with about our feelings. People are not as resilient as we would all like to believe. People don't always recover.

I am reminded of so many children's painful accounts of events in their little lives. Their little hearts are broken. Clearly, they are wounded and damaged. My responses to these little people was to try to plant a seed or two that they could hang onto, and hope that someone after me would come along and water that seed, in order for them to heal. Some days, this just feels like fantasyland to me..."magical thinking."

We are taught as children that if we touch a hot stove, it will burn us. As adults, we seem to forget that lesson. We continue to cross over lines and violate our boundaries and create a pile of regrets. In fact, creating regrets can become a detour for us, a negative way of dealing with life events and interpersonal relationships. People often promise they will change and not do it anymore, but it just isn't that easy...In fact, that is a description of the cycle of domestic violence.

Most people are concerned on a daily basis with making it to work on time, getting their children to school, making sure the bills are paid, putting food on the table, keeping dentist and doctor appointments and getting the dog to the groomer.

We are not focused on "self-actualization," the term coined by the psychologist, Abraham Maslow, who used it to describe a person who is not primarily caught up in maintaining daily chores but rather is committed to the person they want to be and the quality of their relationships. They also concentrate on not engaging in behaviors they will regret. Maslow never found an actualized person under the age of 50.

Regardless of what kind of hand you or I were dealt, or whether or not we are in the minority who can commit to self-actualization, we must focus on where our journey is taking us, no matter what. We need to think about the life we are leading, how it affects the people around us, and how we are going to feel about it when we come to the end. I think this is as good as it gets!

When my oldest son was about seven years old, he and I were walking across a University campus when he asked me what I wanted to be when I grew up. I was about a year away from completing my first Ph.D. and I explained to him what I was studying and why. Then he asked me another question. He asked me what I thought he should be when he grew up. I looked at him and said, "I want you to grow up to be yourself." In other words, I wanted to affirm him and communicate to him that he could be anyone he decided to be.

We don't have to be educated, rich or brilliant to make decisions that will not lead us to regret. We need to be aware of making our own personal journey the best it can be, even though none of us know what is down the road ahead of us. We need to be aware and motivated to make the best of it. None of us are going to do it perfectly. Life and relationships will always represent unfinished business. None of us manage it as well as we had hoped. We simply do the best we can, taking one day at a time, simply putting one foot in front of the other and trusting the ground to be there.

Regrets do not have to ruin our lives. Everyone has crises, problems and sometimes heart-breaking events happen to them. This is the human condition. We need to prepare ourselves, in advance, as best we can. If we are always focused on honoring our own journey, it will make it a little easier. One thing is certain, the more tools we have in our mental health kit, the better are our chances of getting through it and moving forward.

I could not even begin to describe to you the angst I have observed in violent inmates who will never again experience freedom. Some of them are truly remorseful for their behavior which put them there. Nonetheless, they will pay for it for the rest of their lives. These people are often living in their own private hell. They carry burdens which are nearly unfathomable. I recall one inmate who had a commendation in his file from the USA President, but he was serving a life sentence for sexual assault on a child. Again, knowing isn't doing.

Those of us who live in freedom likely underestimate the incredible opportunities to make something wonderful of our lives. What an incredible opportunity we have, until we don't have it anymore....Many of us live as though we are never going to run out of chances to do what we say is important to us.......but it just isn't so. Life is now, always now.

A life filled with regrets is a tough life to lead. If we don't honor our own path, then our journey is going to be a very long and difficult one. We must remember that we are our choices. None of us have a perfect life but we can make it as good as we are able, and be able to take pride in ourselves. We must make the choices we can live with and not regret.

What is there that teaches us to take pride in ourselves? The new normal seems to be teaching us to be clever, be funny, be manipulative, be controlling, get away with as much as we can. "Keep your friends close and your enemies closer." Ours is not a healthy society. What are we teaching our children? We must do the right things for the right reasons to honor our journey is not a popular concept these days. It is all about getting ahead and being 'first.'

If we need to be liked by everyone, we can hardly be concerned with honoring our own journey. We are too busy trying to manipulate everyone around us in order to be liked. This is, indeed, an available choice to us all but I don't see it yielding positive results.

The subject of regrets must include some discussion about grieving. I believe we grieve to the extent that we have loved. We grieve over what we can't change and what we can't get others to change. The truth is that sometimes we simply can't find the peace we are seeking to comfort us.

"If only...." is the message playing in our heads. Sometimes we have to find a way to live with our demons. I think I learned this from the inmates. Perhaps there is a way to carry the grief without the rage. However, if I were a parent of the Sandy Hook Elementary School massacre or the Columbine High School student massacre, I would be hard put to come up with a way to carry the grief without the rage.

My point is that I believe there are some regrets we may never get over. We must be realistic about our expectations of ourselves and others as we get our brains around this kind of a reality. People are damaged.

Speaking of reality, I have been up close and personal with both the victims and the victimizers. Both suffer regrets! Children who are touched wrong, people who are raped, humiliated, bullied, made fun of, special needs students who kill themselves.....many who simply just cannot cope.

It makes me think of a sweatshirt I saw, "Please don't shoot; I'm already wounded." Perhaps most of us sometimes feel as though we are among the walking wounded. Why don't others regret the pain they have caused us?

This Christmas weekend, there were 12 fatalities in Chicago and another 28 wounded from guns. This has been the deadliest year on record of violence in that city. What are we thinking? What are we doing? What are we modeling for our children?

Think about your lifeline. Where do you think you are, at what point? How close do you think you are to the end? Carrie Fisher was 15 minutes from landing at LAX, after a nine hour flight, suffered a cardiac arrest and died 4 days later at the age of 60 with big plans ahead of her. We never know when our time is up, when we run out of time to do what we can about the plans or the regrets in our lives.

Consider your regrets. Can you make any amends? Do you need to express to anyone genuine regret for your actions? Forgiveness can be a balm to relationships and to one's psyche. It can be very healing and bring emotional relief. I believe it is part of mental health to have the ability to acknowledge we made a mistake, own it and apologize for it. What the recipient does with it is on them. We are only responsible for our part.

"I'm sorry" can be two of the most powerful words on the planet. I don't think we hear them nearly enough. Sometime we need to say them to ourselves. Self-forgiveness in an important piece of mental health, maybe the hardest of all.

None of know what is facing us for the rest of our lives. There are likely some surprises for all of us. Nonetheless, if we are committed to honoring our own journey, then we apply the tools we have and use them to do the best we can. None of us are perfect. Regrets are part of everyone's life.

My adult son recently told me his goal in life is to keep his regrets to a minimum. This is a wise goal. The challenging part, however, is making it happen, because knowing isn't doing.

I believe regrets are not unlike unfinished business which weighs us down and interferes with our goals. If our goal is really to honor our own journey, then we need to be aware and think carefully about what we are doing and the impact it is having on us and on the people around us.

Contemplate it.

Be honest with yourself.

Make a decision.

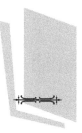

1. Identify your regrets.

2. Be creative in thinking of things you might do to deal with your regrets, e.g., apologize.

3. Raise your sensitivity to your own behaviors so that you don't continue to create regrets.

Chapter Seven

OWNING YOUR LIFE

"Then there was.....you...."

You are unique. In all the world, there is no one else quite like you.

You have unique DNA and your experiences in life are unlike anyone else's. Your brain is arranged in a unique way, based on your experiences, interpretations and choices. You are one of a kind! You have a unique skill set!

I once made a new friend who shared with me, after we had several meetings together, "You really don't appear to care what people think of you." My response was to humbly reply that I had worked for a very long time to be the person I have become and I can't afford to let others' praise or blame be a guide for my life. People who know me best say I am a "What you see is what you get kind of person." Actually, I believe that is accurate and that it has served me well in my profession. If I was dependent on likeability from others, I couldn't have done by job given that I have spent a lifetime telling people things they don't want to hear.

One of the biggest challenges to mental health that I am aware of is helping people to value themselves. I'm not talking about narcissism or arrogance. Rather, I'm referring to a genuine belief in the person who is aware of their gifts and strengths. They are also aware of their need to make improvements, and believe they can!

The reason I believe healthy self-esteem is so important is because it is the springboard for affirming others, especially the people we live with under our own roof.

If you don't think well of yourself, you are unlikely to be affirming the people around you because you simply don't have that gift to give. It has taken me a very long time to figure this out.

I have spent a lifetime needing and trying to get affirmation from people who simply didn't have it to give. It wasn't about me. If you don't think well of yourself, you are unlikely to be able to affirm those around you. The better you feel about yourself, the more likely you are to build others up rather than tear them down. We find what we're looking for. If we want to see the weaknesses in a person, then that's what we'll see. If we look for something positive, we can usually find it and reinforce it. If the world would function at this level, we would be living in a very different kind of world. This is why parents and teachers are so critical. They have the power to make a difference. It is also what makes so many grandmothers special to so many children.

According to the psychologists who have constructed Theories of Personality, they believe personality is basically set by the age of five. They also know that self-esteem is very resistant to change. It is not impossible, but it is rare.

It is a very long road to improving self-esteem. How much easier to take the time and effort to build up our young people from an early age, to affirm their strengths and encourage them at a very early age.

It is easier to fix a broken child than a broken adult, but my experience has been that it is nearly impossible to do either.

While I was a college professor, I conducted an exercise, asking students to write down three positive and three negative things about themselves. The negatives came quickly but many of them still couldn't come up with three positive attributes, even after ten minutes. These were college students. What does this tell us? Out of the 65 students in the class, only five of them said they would want to be born into the family they were if, in fact, they would have had a choice. These are disturbing statistics.

It is my belief that one of the fundamentals of mental health is the need to believe in and think well of oneself. Another is the ability to block. Another is to understand that the things people say about you really says more about them than you. Just learning and applying these three simple concepts can change lives.

It is simply not true that "sticks and stone may break your bones but words can never harm you." We should stop teaching that lie to our children. Nothing could be further from the truth. I have treated seniors in their 70's and 80's who are still struggling with things said to them during their childhood.

My point here is that it is very hard to own who we are or how much confidence we have in the path we are on if we continually keep giving away our power and allow others to take control of our journey. If we give a horse its reins, it will head for the barn every time. We must take control if we expect to come to the end of our lives in a place and at a point that will enable us to get go, with peace and a sense of fulfillment.

So often we become intimidated by others' opinions of us. If someone doesn't like us, there may be a million reasons why. I know I don't have the time or energy to contemplate all of them. I believe we need to follow our heart, be our own person and let the chips fall where they will.

The blatant reality is that not everyone is going to like us. If we need that, then we best never open our mouths, be honest or take any risks. It's that simple. People don't even need a reason not to like someone. It's just the way it is. We can learn from those people and profit from their feedback but we better think twice before we relinquish our power to them. We need to be authentically who we are. That is the shape of owning our unique journey.

All of our paths include negatives and positives. It includes accepting, maybe even cherishing, certain parts of ourselves while we loathe other parts. This, I believe, is the human condition. The truth is, however, that we have to embrace and accept all the parts and pieces of ourselves before we can take measures to change. In other words, we need to own our path before we can navigate it to change directions. If we are in denial about our journey, we will likely never make the changes because we won't even realize they exist.

Owning one's journey can take many different forms. Ideally, the ownership of one's personal path is to accept the challenge to make it as good as we are capable so that we can transition to a peaceful ending.

Speaking positively, children and adults can be taught to be all they can be. They can make changes, but we don't seem to realize our time constraints. We just don't have forever to make them happen.

In my young life, I lost several people to death, which had a huge impact on me. I experienced loss at an early age, before I had any tools to cope with them. This was extremely painful.

The upside, however, is that I became aware at an early age that people are not for forever. I have short life lines in my family.

Ultimately, no one but us can decide our path. It is up to us. When we come to the end of our lives, we will have to take full responsibility for whoever we turned out to be. Our chance to do that will not last forever. We need to focus on what's between the dash of when we were born and when we die.

2016 has been a year of loss--of movie stars and well-known people, and too many tragedies. Just this week, there was a fire which took the lives of 36 people, the youngest just 17. Many of them texted loved-ones, telling them they were going to die. Yet, they had come to that place for a celebration. We never know when our time has come to an end. This is actually a profound reality, something us humans seem to work overtime to deny. No one wants to think about death and dying. Yet it is a very big part of life.

On a personal note, what three words might you or I use to describe ourselves? And, which three words would we like to believe others would use to describe us after we leave the Earth? We can pick out one of these words and work on having that quality in our life. We can put a foundation under it and make it happen. "Yes we can." No matter what it is, we can work on it and attain it. Believe it!

Human beings are very powerful and can accomplish great things. There exist remarkable human beings all around us. You are one of them.

You were created in the image of God. You have special gifts and abilities which were intended for you to use, not ignore or abuse. You have the ability to bless others with your gifts. Believe it.

A good skill to have is the ability to think outside the box in order to get to where we want to be. Sometimes we have to take risks in order to get there. We have to believe it is possible to reach our goals.

We can't afford to procrastinate, get depressed or give up. There is already way too much of this in the world.

We all need to look for ways to speak our truth in love and make it matter, at least to ourselves. We need to nurture and hold our beliefs dear and stay committed to them throughout our life.

We need to keep the challenge of balance in our lives as steady and beautiful as we possibly can, with a belief in ourselves and in our world that can never be destroyed. We need to own our balance with a vengeance and not let anyone pull us off our path.

We are, of course, talking about the process of owning and honoring our own very personal journey.

We can do this. We can be this!

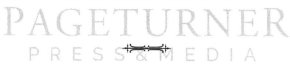

1. What three words would you use to describe yourself?

2. Think about making a change that you could help make in someone else's life.

3. Dare to dream of something you want to accomplish. Put the foundation under your plans and make it happen.

Chapter Eight

FINDING THE BALANCE

"If only I may grow--firmer,
simpler, quieter, warmer."
(Dag Hammarsjold)

Some might argue that finding the balance is a myth, a fairytale. It's like the 'impossible dream.'

Remember the movie, "The Karate Kid, when Daniel was constantly encouraged by his trainer to find the balance. Would most of us even recognize it if we found it? There is so much that competes for our attention.

Also, the balance probably looks very different to each one of us. What works for one doesn't necessarily work for another. We each have to find it for ourselves. How do we do it with all of the pressures we all face? When do we even find time for ourselves, let alone the balance?....all good questions....

Most of us weren't born into a family of movie stars, didn't get chosen to play for the NFL, didn't make the cut for Miss America, didn't get a trust fund, etc.

Although we look at those people with envy, they have their challenges as well. Have you noticed how tragically some of their lives have ended? Money, fame and drugs aren't all they're cracked up to be. Look around. There are so many examples of tragic endings of famous people. Just because someone catches a break and ends up with fame and money doesn't mean they are applying healthy rules for life and well-being. Winners of large lotteries also fall into that category.

No matter who we are, the gifts and talents we bring to the table, the challenge is to make the best of it, whatever that needs to mean. Probably the best thing we can do is to take the very best care of ourselves so the people we love most don't have to. Self-care is a beautiful example of healthy self-esteem and honoring our journey.

In addition to healthy physical care, we would all do well to pay attention to our mental health. This is actually harder. In short, it means staying off detours, being able to block, reframing every day, making healthy choices, affirming others, maintaining self-esteem and trying hard to be the best possible person we can be every day of our lives. This is hard work.

As a matter of fact, I have felt somewhat overwhelmed this week with trying to maintain my balance as I deal with serious issues of people I care about. Medical crises tend to leave me feeling raw and unprepared. I hate them and I don't manage them well, partly because of my long history in dealing with medical crises and death. It reinforces my understanding of wanting to numb out, to slip onto a detour that will deter the pain. I won't let it happen, but I'd be less than honest if I didn't admit that I'm tempted. Battles are won and lost in the mind which drives our choices and how we cope with it all.

Mental health demands focus, as does balance. I have actually drawn a path which represents my life; then I have drawn all the detoursvI have taken to avoid the pain of the paths. I've been surprised to discover so many of them. The detours are tenacious. They can be dangerous. They are always a bad choice.

Staying aware and being honest with ourselves, no matter what kind of a day we are having, is very important. It must be from real honesty that we make our best choices, even the painful ones.

The recent death of Carrie Fisher caught my attention as I was hearing about something she said. She said she recalled, as a child, having her nose pressed up against the window of the bakery, but felt like a loaf of bread inside. As an adult, she relayed to a famous friend that when your heart is broken, you need to find a way to turn it into art.

These are mysterious words and, truth bebknown, we all have that deeper side of ourselves that we rarely share with anyone. Maybe that's why they invented mental health workers.

I believe Carrie Fisher is an amazing example of a woman who was dealt a difficult hand with special challenges and was born into a divided family with famous parents, addictions, rehab, etc. It appears she never gave up. She used her incredible abilities to make the best possible life for herself. This is what I'm talking about.

It has been several years now since my accident in the work place which ended my career. My life, since then, has become a lot about pain management. It is never a space I anticipated. My inner dialogue tells me, "That was my life then, this is my life now. Live it." We can probably all relate to that message. All of us have highs and lows and we can rarely anticipate when or how it will change. If only someone had some magic to make it all go back to the way it used to be. If we could just do a rewind! It isn't going to happen. It was what it was, and it is what it is. There is no place for magical thinking.

I once asked my Mother what she would change in her life if given the chance. I was shocked by her answer. She simply said, "Nothing." I took that to mean that in spite of all the trauma and sadness in her life, it brought her to the beautiful person and Mother she turned out to be. She was one of the greatest influences and blessings of my life. She was my friend in the family. She was the wind beneath my wings.

So, finding the balance includes acceptance of everything in our life that has ever happened to us. This includes learning to reframe certain parts, and keep moving forward, avoiding the detours. I think it's rather like learning to ride a bicycle. It gets easier, until it gets harder... We can't afford to get bogged down in "Why?" or the "What ifs....?" It is what it is.

Everyone walks with a limp. Everyone has pain and issues they are working on. Usually, the rest of us are clueless about it. People tend not to show their vulnerabilities. It doesn't feel safe (and probably isn't). We all live with our skeletons and demons and work at keeping them hidden. This can be part of our version of balance, although there are probably at least a million things that can throw all of us off our balance. It is a daily challenge.

One of the reasons I journal is to use it as a means of helping me keep my balance. It is kind of like having a mirror held up in front of me that never lies to me. It helps me see things more clearly and helps me to be aware of what I need to be working on. It shows me where I am off balance, whether I want to see it or not.

I have to remind myself, from time to time, that the mirror is my friend, not my enemy. Even so, some days, I know I resent it!

Finding and maintaining the balance requires courage, honesty and a real desire to live our best life. I work every day to find the balance and some days, I can't. Other days, it seems to reach out to me like a good friend and invites me to follow it. Clearly, it is an unending adventure and challenge.

One of my struggles includes staying off the detour of resentment. If I'm not careful, I find myself ruminating over things I simply must let go of because I'll never be able to change them. Just because people are related does not make them relatable or close friends. Letting go is a must of mental health. That task is clearly mine and one I must find a way to do if I want to have balance in my life. These are not easy challenges.

Part of balance has to do with risk. If we don't want to get hurt, then we shouldn't take any risks. They say that a risk is a win but it certainly doesn't always feel that way. On a positive note, I know that when my feelings are hurt, it is an opportunity for me to learn more about myself. I must maintain this focus in order to be focused, healthy and balanced, a hard lesson to learn

Dr. Leon Fine, a psychologist, made a thoughtful remark. He said,

"Only by risking can I get rewarded; by risking I might get hurt. By not risking, I get neither rewarded nor hurt; I merely hurt quietly."

Too many are hurting quietly. Don't be one of them.

Balance can be a goal, in some form, for all of us, no matter what challenges we face in our lives. Paying attention to our boundaries can help us. Violating our personal boundaries takes us to detours which often lead to many other problems. We really need to understand our vulnerabilities.

I have come to realize that my defenses are not as strong as they once were and that I have suffered what I call 'vicarious post-traumatic stress' from my work. It has impacted my life in very painful ways. I do what I can but I really know "I can't fix it," although I have spent a life time trying to do exactly that.

Balance is our friend. We need to look for it and welcome it into our lives.

Speaking of balance, in the many months I have now spent here working on this book, my goals have boiled down to only three. Many days they look unattainable and my attitude is less than what I would like for it to be. Nonetheless, it is what it is. I refuse to give up although if I'm honest I must say I am tempted at times to do exactly that. Balancing my personal physical pain with major goals has turned out to be a very big hill for me to climb. I am who I am and can do what I can. That is the shape of acceptance and balance for me. That is the shape of honoring my journey.

We must believe in the balance and encourage ourselves as we seek to live it out in our daily lives. To make this even more real to myself, I did an exercise the other day. I wrote my obituary, not to be morbid but simply to see what I would say about myself. It was actually quite enlightening, humbling and actually made me smile, when I read: "She gave at the office!:-)"

If you're up for a big dose of reality, try it! You may learn something new about yourself. You may even be encouraged to figure out and work on the shape of balance in your own life, maybe even become motivated to make some changes.

Go for it!

1. Identify a change you could make in your life that would give it greater balance.

2. Identify alternative changes that would make your life happier.

3. Start today by including a positive change for yourself.

Chapter Nine

KEEPING IT REAL

"As a man thinks in his heart....so is he....."

There are two distinct levels in keeping it real: one is interpersonal, the other is intrapersonal.

Our own internal mental mechanism of how we process our thoughts is critical in how we relate to others and how we live out our lives. It guides our choices.

What we filter out from our thoughts and share with others is a special process that shapes our lives. Certainly, it shapes how others receive us and think of us; also, how we think of ourselves.

While everyone has a need to be liked, I believe we need to be careful to not placate our integrity for the sake of likeability.

Keeping it real was a theme in a course I taught at a Level 4 prison. Inmates have little use for trivia and untruths. They seem to be able to spot a phony in an instant. They have little tolerance for being told less than the truth. They appear to be in that 4 1/2 % of people who keep it real and tell it like it is. This, in fact, is a lifestyle for many of them. I came to appreciate it and to emulate it. I realized I could be shredded in half a second if I presented anything that was less than trustworthy. This was valuable learning for me.

I came to respect and practice keeping it real in that environment, and in every environment.

I also recall, during my training as a psychologist, when I first visited an Alcohol

Anonymous meeting (AA). I was amazed and completely impressed with the level of honesty I heard there. It was entirely refreshing to me. I admired the level of self-disclosure and the honesty I witnessed. I wished I could take it with me and spread it around the world. I felt completely comfortable. I was amazed. Somehow, pain has a way of cutting through the superficial, enabling us to reach our core and bare our soul.

When we keep it real, we are being authentic, to ourselves and to the people we rub elbows with every day. Actually, trust is very related to keeping it real. We tend to trust people we perceive as authentic. I also think we tend to trust ourselves the most when we learn to be brutally honest with ourselves. Other people notice that quality too, and are often drawn to it.

Aren't we all tired of being told some version of the truth, something which undermines our trust in the person who functions that way, especially if they live under our own roof? Over time, we pull away from these people, sometimes unconsciously. But, if we decide to get honest about our feelings, we know that we do not trust certain people, often for reasons of which we are unsure. It is simply intuitive. Sadly, this describes the way I have heard many children describe their feelings about their parents.

Pretenses about most anything in our life does not serve us well. It does not serve parenting well. It does not serve marriage or relationships well in enabling people to bond. In fact, it does not serve anyone well.

We need to know who we are and present that self in our everyday life. I don't believe we respect ourselves more when we are less than honest with ourselves or with others.

A very long time ago I had someone challenge me to be "brutally honest" about myself and my life. I accepted that challenge, reluctantly I'm sure, but I've never forgotten it. It was some of the best advice I ever received.

We distrust people who aren't honest with us and everyone seems to know implicitly who these people are, although some people seem to be masters of deception. I've met some of them. Don't we want to disengage from them as quickly as possible? It is not so easy to do!

There are times when I find I can't hardly stand myself when I am around certain people. In fact, I remember saying to someone once, "I can't stand me when I'm around you." That is no way to live, especially when it is someone you live with under the same roof. That had to change, and did.

Part of honoring our journey is being genuinely authentic, telling it like it is, inviting others to develop a relationship with us which is founded on trust, not lies, or alcohol, or drugs, or hidden agendas or being used, or on detours.

We can't expect to grow in our self esteem if we keep presenting ourselves as someone we know we are not. That will never work for us, or for them. Being a phony will ultimately kill you.

Successful marriages, families, parent-child relationships, the fiber of the family has to be built on truths we can take to the bank.

We have to stop thinking that we aren't good enough to share the truth about ourselves. We must stop making up stories that make us seem better than we are. It's O.K. to admit that we failed, that we didn't do our best or try our hardest. We are best served by admitting mistakes, being honest about them, and being determined to do better next time. I believe that's what moving forward really means when it comes to honoring our journey. We need to model this for our children.

When we do something that disappoints us about ourselves, we need to be able to separate our what we DO from who we ARE. We can hate the behaviors and still have love for the person. We need to learn to separate behaviors from the core of the person.

The truth of the matter is, "I can't be right for you if I'm not right for me." People, I believe, need to spend more time thinking about their true integrity and make it important to them. This is one of the ways we maintain self-esteem. If we start giving away pieces of ourselves, we may wake up one day and have difficulty rounding up all of our parts. Some we may never get back.

I remember once telling someone, "I can't be that for you because that isn't who I am." When we get that honest, we are doing actual negotiating about the viability of building a trusting relationship. It is better to admit early on who we are and who we aren't in honest ways, rather than find it out later. This could help avoid a world of heartache.

There is a definite challenge in balancing integrity with honesty. Of course, it would not be wise to simply let everything we are thinking slip off of our tongue. There are ways to express thoughts and ways not to express them. Speaking the truth in love appears to be a good guideline for communicating.

How we act this out at home creates powerful modeling for children. It shows them an example of how life is to be done. I recall an incident where the teenager heard his father tell his wife to only claim those items on the tax return that could be traced back to them. Clearly, this was an expression of fraud that could be interpreted as the way to prepare your tax returns, or for that matter, how to live life in general. In other words, the message isn't "Don't cheat." The message is "Don't cheat and get caught."

I once asked my adult children the lessons they had learned as children from their parents. Their answers were thoughtful and interesting. We need to be aware of the influence we are having on the people around us by the things we say and do. Even more importantly, we need to be aware of how our presentation of self influences our own self-esteem. We need to be making choices we can live with and be at peace.

Keeping it real doesn't imply that we need to go around hurting everyone's feelings so that we can feel good about ourselves. It does, however, imply that we have a responsibility to be "congruent," that our actions and our behavior are consistent. It is when we think one thing and say or do another that it becomes a problem.

A well-known psychologist, Dr. Carl Rogers, said that it never pays in the long run to behave as though we are someone we are not. This does not contribute to our mental health. In fact, that kind of lifestyle can easily turn onto a detour which we may not even realize we are on until it's too late to retreat from it.

As I have continually stated, you have to like yourself in order to honor your journey. In fact, a way to start honoring it is to change the things you don't like or respect about yourself.

I have had many people tell me things about themselves (who weren't my patients) and swore me to secrecy to never tell anyone. If we're doing things and don't want others to know, maybe that's a sign that we need to rethink our behaviors.

The key, I believe, to keeping it real lies within our intrapersonal processes. I think we are wise to be brutally honest with ourselves, then figure out how we want to parse out that honesty. No matter what, it should be some form of speaking our truth in an appropriate way. Otherwise, we spend our lives not only not honoring our journey, but defiling it, giving us more to feel regretful about in the end.

Since I began this project and have committed to spending this year on this project, I have had a lot of time to think. That fact, along with all of the journaling I have been doing, has led me into some painful truths about myself and my relationships that I did not see coming.

Since I've been here, I have made a definite curve in the road of my life which I have found painful, but healthy and real. I can't honestly say that I always enjoy keeping it real. Sometimes, that is simply a gateway to some kind of personal pain. Nonetheless, I believe it is vital to honoring my journey.

My closest friends have passed away. I miss them more than I can say as they were my lighthouses, my sounding boards, my reality checks, and more. Since I am the youngest person in my family of five, I am one of two left. I'm not sure I like being the youngest. I see what is coming.

While I believe children are an incredible gift, the parent-child relationships ends in adulthood and what is left is not always bonding. This can be painful, but better than kidding oneself.

There is so very much for which I am grateful. In the same breath, I can admit I would not wish my life on anyone. Yet, I believe it was the 'exam' that was meant for me and I am committed to staying focused on service, hope and compassion, no matter what.

So, I encourage you to honor your journey and your passion with honesty, integrity and peace. You are the only one who can.

---

1. What area of your life do you have the most difficulty keeping it real?

2. Is there a specific person you need or want to have a conversation with and express your feelings, whatever they may be?

3. What would bring you relief and joy in your life as you think about keeping it real as you honor your journey?

Chapter Ten

PURSUING PEACE

"Be careful what you think for
your thoughts guard your life."
(Proverbs 4:23)

Our thoughts control our lives through our choices! Sometimes they guard us. At other times, they make us vulnerable.

"Everyone has their own version of reality." For example, I do not assume, for example, that my Christian beliefs are shared by all of my readers. Nonetheless, I feel the need and desire to share what brings me peace.

No matter who we are, what our issues and belief system are, we can pursue peace. However, I have found that it will usually entail some form of letting go.

As I consider this process in my own life, I am strongly challenged by my own personal collection of regrets, pain, failures, resentments, post-traumatic-stress events, wrongs that will never be made right, and so many other issues that are detours to my peace. Continually, I look for ways to let them go. I think we must let go of what we cannot change. The bell has rung, we can't un-ring it. That ship has sailed.

"I have discovered that my faith is seeing light and hope with my heart when all my eyes see is darkness. "

I feel blessed to have been given the gift of faith in God and believe this has made all the difference in my life, yet I am clear that not everyone shares this point of view!

For as far back as I can remember, I grew up knowing I wanted to accomplish certain things. I wanted to go to college, but no one in my family of five ever did. There was no money to send me to college. I was the youngest. My Mother didn't finish high school, due to some very sad circumstances in her life, and my Father was disabled in a horrible accident when I was seven years old. Both of my parents lost a parent when they were children. I had dreams. I wanted to adopt a child but was actually surprised when it happened. I wanted to get a Ph.D. and try to make some kind of positive contribution to the world. I ended up with 4 college degrees, including two Ph.D.'s. My point here is not to be bragging, but rather to make the point that if we don't dream and envision what we really want our life to be, we are less likely to achieve those things.

We have to believe in the possibilities we care about and develop the attitude of "Yes I can." I feel so indebted to the people who believed in me along the way and helped me realize my dreams were reachable and could become a reality. They are my heroes.

We have to plant dream seeds and water them every day of our lives. We have to believe in ourselves.

If I can do it, anyone can!

While I champion positive thinking and living, I don't always model it or experience it. While I struggle to get go of traumatic memories and look for ways to rid myself of what I call 'vicarious trauma,' it still troubles me at times. While I have worked throughout my life to come to terms with various forms of trauma, I am not always able to do it. I find this to be an unending challenge and so I am constantly working to find ways to let go of what I cannot change. My dreams frequently remind me of my struggles.

This is one of the hardest things I've ever had to do. I wrestle with issues of rage and anger for experiences I have witnessed personally. I have seen evil up close and personal and it has had a profound impact on my life.

In spite of the issues with which we struggle and have difficulty shedding, I believe that at the end of the day (and the end of life), that my personal faith in a wise and loving Creator is the foundation and strength of my life. He is the Source of my peace. He IS Peace.

This is the reason I chose and practiced my profession. My faith is the reason I continue to write books. My faith is what gets me out of bed each day. My faith is the reason I keep trying to make a difference for good. My faith is the reason I continue to care.

To be clear, I am not talking about 'religion.' (I think I grew up attending the First Church of the Neurotic!) I have actually come to loathe most of the religious experiences of my life. I believe they were largely deceptive.

I think I used to believe that Jesus would love me more because of my list of do's and don'ts, rights and wrongs that I was so careful to follow. I was steeped in legalism. How totally misled I was. I was like a Pharisee. It took me a lifetime to sort out the difference between religion and true spiritual relational faith in a loving, omnipotent God.

I am talking about a personal relationship with a living, loving, dynamic, all-knowing God who created human beings and has a purpose for every human life. It is what challenges me constantly to do and strive to be my best and know that I am loved unconditionally, whether I feel it or not. What does your belief system tell you and how is it working for you?

If one takes my point of view, then the goal becomes that of seeking to fulfill the plan and purpose for my life, to even believe that one exists. Scripture declares that before we were even born, God saw us in our Mother's womb and scheduled every day of our lives! (Psa. 139).

I have found this especially challenging as I review my personal experiences in working with devastated others, both children and adults. How is it that a loving God would allow so much suffering? My answer is that I don't have a clue.

I have simple faith that He is the God of the Universe and it is my job to maintain my simple faith that He knows what He is doing, whether I understand it or not. In the meantime, my heart breaks for those people, the children especially, who have been so traumatically brutalized. I can't even find the words to describe my feelings.

Finding peace in our world today is a major challenge. There is so much violence in the world. Without faith, I would have great difficulty facing it. Scripture has endless verses regarding peace:

Jesus identified Himself as the "Prince of Peace." We are encouraged to "Let nothing disturb your peace." How to practice these truths on a daily basis remains a challenge for me. I simply know the bottom line is that my faith in a loving God who created us in His image has a positive plan for our lives, whether we feel it or believe it or not.

We are loved unconditionally by the One Who says He will never leave us nor forsake us. We are empowered and receive our strength from a forgiving God who only wants the best for us, who sticks closer to us than a brother.

Perhaps my friend and theologian, Dr. Haddon Robinson, said it best:

"Whole faith in a Sovereign God enables us to trust when we cannot trace, step when we cannot see, and undergo what we may not understand."

When our challenges and struggles have come to an end, no matter what our life has been, we can take our last breath in peace as we cross over into the loving arms of our beloved Creator.

1. What is your personal belief system?

2. How does it impact your life?

3. Are there any changes you need to make? If so, what are they and how are you going to make them a reality while you still can?

EPILOGUE

The writing of this book has been very challenging for me.

It has been an effort at balance -- being helpful, of applying principles that I've learned through formal education, but mostly from my time in the trenches with the unlovely...the abused and hurting, the wounded, the mentally ill, the hated, and the forgotten. I feel as though I have lived a lifetime with those people. They have become a part of me.

I sought to strike a balance of presenting my own private belief system with the understanding that not all readers would agree with me. My intent was never to force my belief system on anyone, but rather to share my personal 'truths,' based on my life experiences. No one, for example, will ever convince me that life is fair.

I worked hard in this book to be honest, yet with integrity--not disclosing anything that was not mine to share. There is so much more I could have said, but suffice it to say, it is what it is. Confidentiality is a bench mark for me and I take it very seriously.

Because of the nature of the topic of this book, it was an effort for me to keep it positive. There were at least a million negative things I left out.

We've all heard enough of what's wrong in the world. My goal was to be positive, to encourage you to take hold of your life and feel empowered to make it whatever you really want it to be. Believe in yourself, set realistic and positive goals you can reach that will make you, and those you love, a happier, more fulfilled person by finding ways to honor your journey.

My ultimate goal was to provide a platform for you to envision making your life what you really want it to be, to believe that it really is a possibility but no one is going to do it for you. You must risk trying. It is work! There are a million stories of famous people who failed dozens of times before their goal was realized. Don't ever give up on your dreams, no matter what! Miracles still happen.

It is my wish that God will richly bless us all as we seek to honor our journey, and our truths.

May we stay off of the detours, learn to reframe and to block, make positive and productive changes, hold our regrets to a minimum and learn to keep it real.

May we know we are loved unconditionally and are not alone, no matter how alone we may feel. May we stay focused, treat ourselves and others with compassion, take risks and find the balance, knowing that we can accomplish great things, and that giving up is never an option.

Let's make it happen!!

Shirley Gilbert sjg11643@yahoo.com

CPSIA information can be obtained
at www.ICGtesting.com
Printed in the USA
BVHW031443291121
622773BV00002B/116